EAT SO WHAT!

SMART WAYS TO STAY HEALTHY

VOLUME 2

I0415198

Nutritional Food Guide for Vegetarians for A Disease Free Healthy Life (Mini Edition)

LA FONCEUR

CONTENTS

CHAPTER 1

10 REASONS YOU SHOULD START EATING ALMONDS EVERY DAY

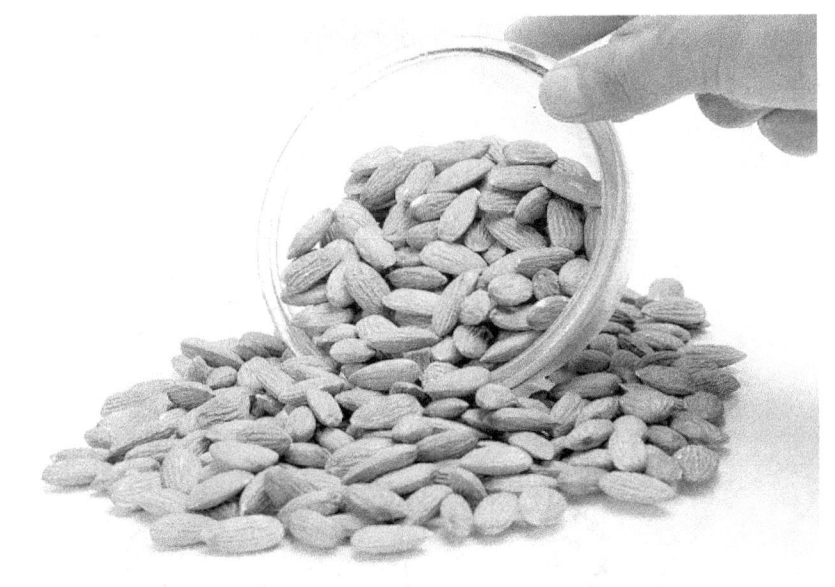

Almonds are among the healthiest of tree nuts. Natural, unsalted almonds are a nutritious snack loaded with minerals with plenty of health benefits. Just a handful of almonds (10-15 kernels) a day helps promote heart health, skin and hair health and prevent weight gain, and it may even help fight diseases like Alzheimer's and diabetes.

Types of almonds:

Bitter: These almonds are used for making (almond) oil, which has multiple benefits.

Sweet: Sweet almonds are edible in nature.

Below are 10 Reasons You Should Start Eating Almonds Every Day:

1. Almonds Improve Skin Health

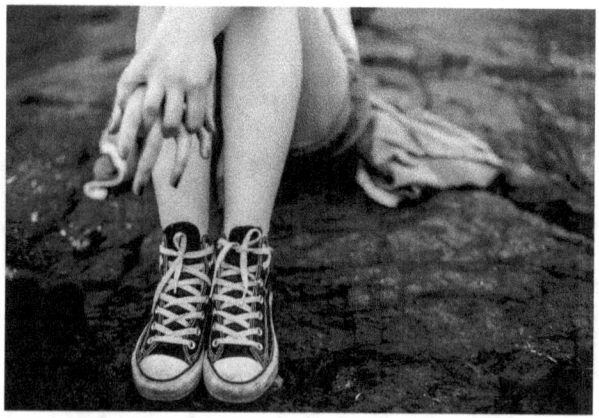

Want to have glowing, healthy skin? Eat almonds! Almonds are a great source of vitamin E and antioxidants, which fight free radicals and reduce inflammation, preserving your skin healthy and young. People with dermatitis problem should eat almonds daily. Antioxidants in almonds can fight the damage produced by UV rays, pollution, and a poor diet on the skin. Almonds fight against aging, malnourished skin and prevent skin cancer.

2. Almonds Maintain a Healthy Brain Function

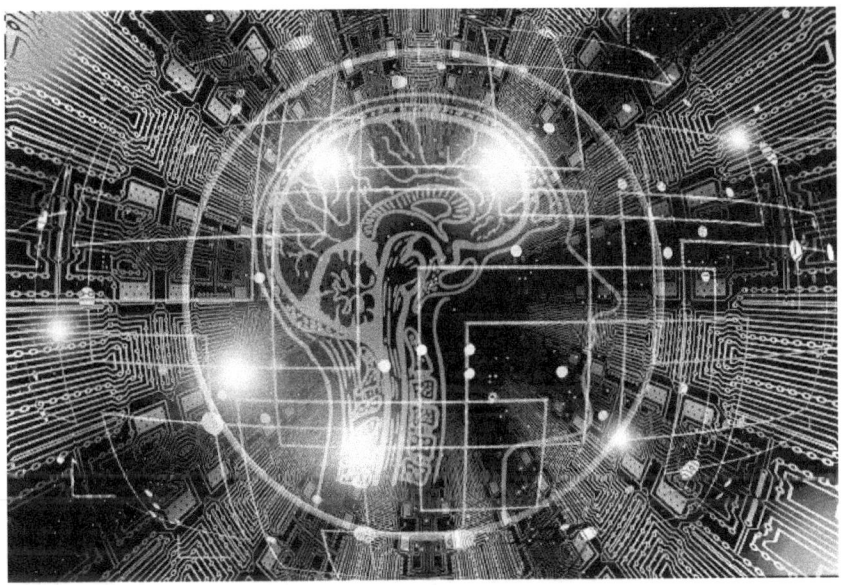

Almonds are rich in riboflavin and L-carnitine. These two substances prevent cognitive decline and support healthy neurological activity, reducing the brain's inflammatory processes. Eating almonds every day can prevent cognitive diseases like dementia and Alzheimer's disease.

3. Almonds Improve Hair Health

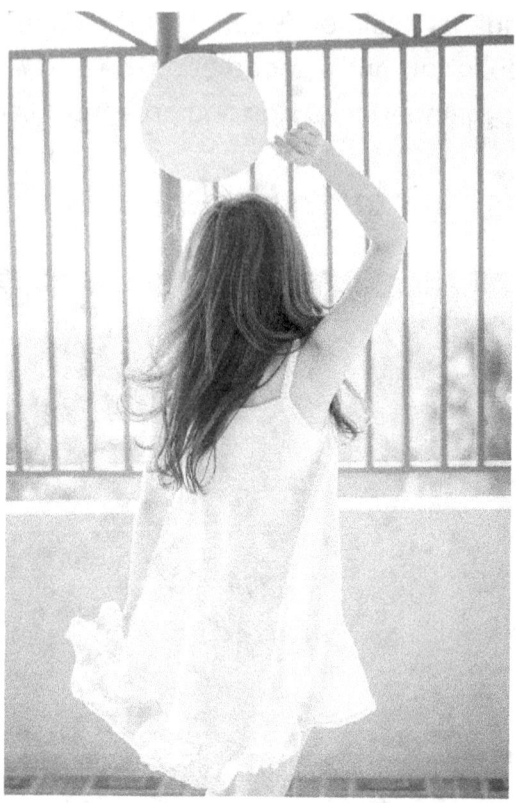

Almonds are absolutely bursting with biotin. A single serving contains over 50 percent of your daily value. Biotin (also known as vitamin H) helps many bodily processes, but perhaps its most prominent role is aiding in healthy hair formation. Biotin deficiency can lead to an unhealthy scalp and brittle, thinning hair. Since just a single serving of almonds contains over half your daily requirement, they're a fantastic food for keeping hair strong, healthy, and beautiful.

Read 10 Most Important Nutrients for Hair Health in the book Secret of Healthy Hair.

4. Almonds Keep Heart Healthy and Prevent Heart Attacks

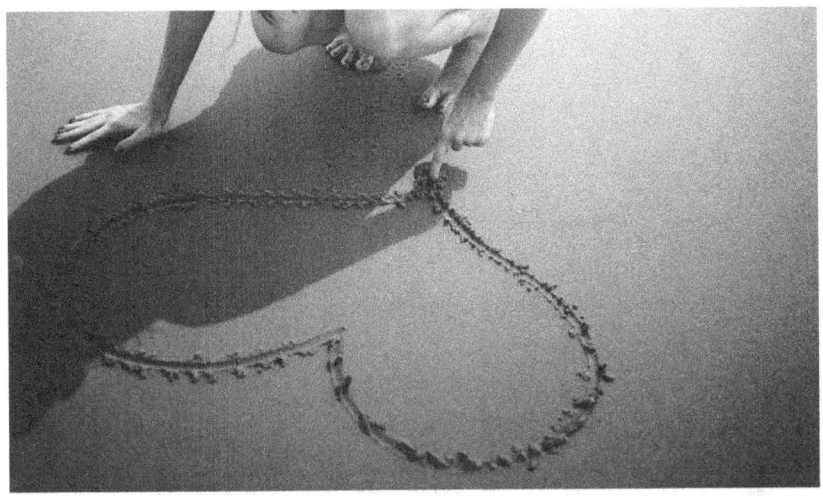

Almonds have high levels of monounsaturated and polyunsaturated fats. Also known as "good fats," they have been shown to have a significant positive impact on cholesterol. A better cholesterol profile greatly reduces the risk of blocked arteries, the biggest culprit behind heart attacks and strokes. Eating more almonds equals a healthier heart.

5. Almonds for Weight Loss

Almonds are packed with a lot of fiber and protein content which takes a longer time to digest, which results in a fuller stomach and lesser cravings. Plus, protein helps in the development of lean muscle mass. Almonds are a perfect low-carb snack and ideal for those who are on a low-carb diet.

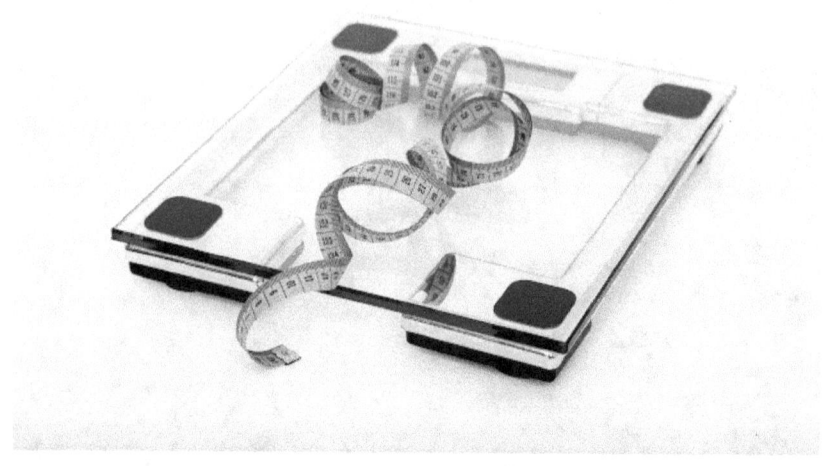

6. Almond Benefits Blood Pressure Levels

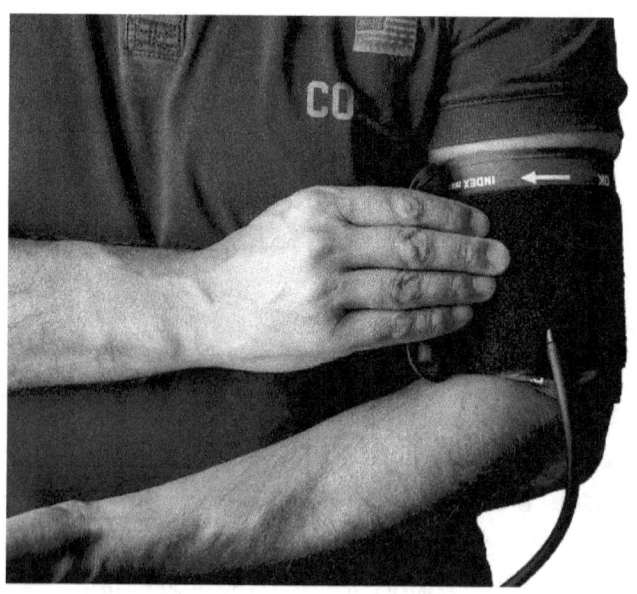

Almonds fend off magnesium deficiency. Magnesium deficiency is strongly linked to high blood pressure. If you do not meet the dietary recommendations for magnesium, adding almonds to your diet could have a huge impact. The magnesium in almonds may help lower blood pressure levels. High blood pressure is one of the leading drivers of heart attacks, strokes, and kidney failure.

7. Almond Increase Digestion and Metabolism

Almonds are good for digestion. Eating almonds could help improve digestive health by increasing levels of beneficial gut bacteria. As well as being high in vitamin E and other minerals, almonds are now believed to increase good bacteria in the gut. Almond milk contains secret traces of fiber. Fiber is known for its digestion-enhancing benefits. Thus, almond milk eases the problem of indigestion largely. Increased digestion flushes unwanted and unhealthy toxins out of the human body system. This further increases the metabolic rate of the human body.

8. Almonds Prevent Cancer

Almonds are an excellent reserve of vitamin E, Phytochemicals, and flavonoids, which control the progression of breast cancer cells. Fibers in almonds help in detoxifying the body. It enables food to move through the digestive system more efficiently. This process cleanses the digestive system, thus lower the risk of colon cancer.

9. Almonds Strengthen Bones and Teeth

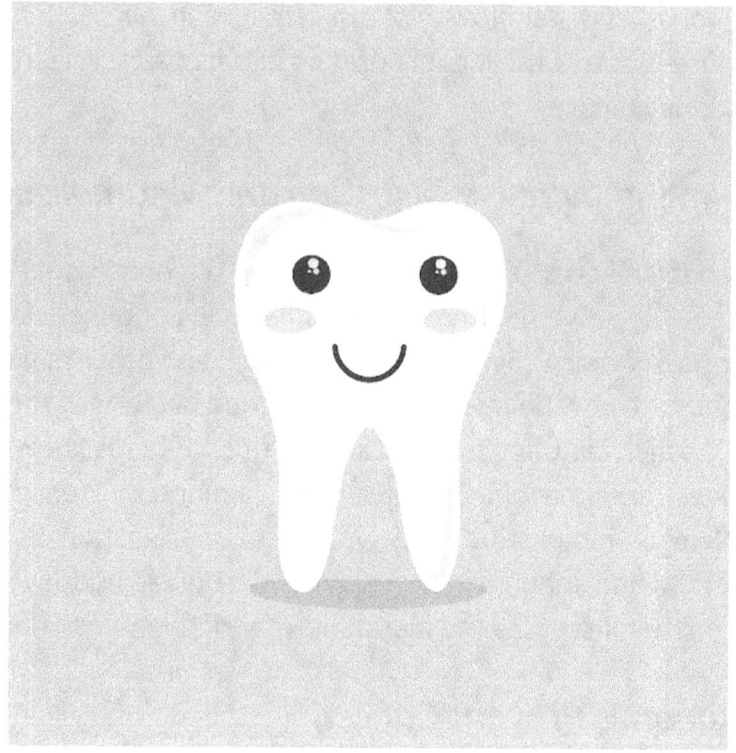

Almonds contain nearly 200 mg of the recommended daily dose of calcium. They also deliver a whole host of nutrients— fiber, manganese, phosphorus, vitamin E, which avert osteoporosis, strengthen teeth, improve bone mineral density, and strengthen the skeletal system.

10. Almonds Prevent Birth Defects

Folic acid in almonds protects the baby while still in the womb from neural tube defects. Folic acid plays a big function in healthy cell growth and tissue configuration, and therefore, it is very important for the fetus's healthy growth. It also helps with the development of the nervous system and the bones.

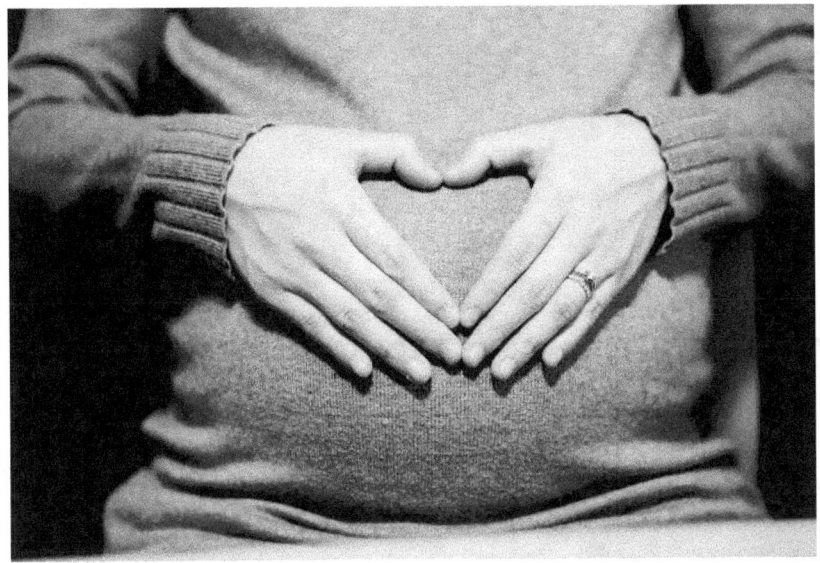

Conclusion

One should eat soaked almonds as soaking almonds neutralize enzyme inhibitors, thus aiding digestion. Soaking almonds help in reducing phytic acids in the outer layer of almonds. The outer layer of bran of almonds can block calcium absorption and affect magnesium, iron, copper, and zinc, which we consume. Soaked almonds have higher B Vitamins. They help in the breakdown of gluten, which neutralizes toxins in colons and makes proteins more available for absorption. It is also to be kept in mind that almonds have calories and hence should be consumed in controlled quantities. Excess consumption of almonds can be bad for the heart as well as your body weight.

CHAPTER 2

10 REASONS WHY ALCOHOL IS A BIG NO NO!!!

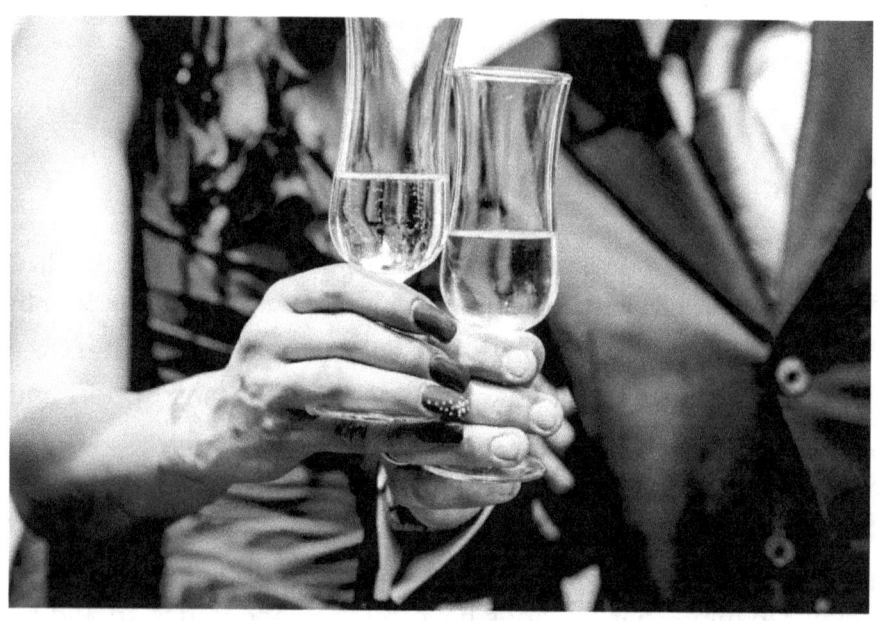

For many people, alcohol consumption has become a part of life. Alcohol is basically a chemical that can damage the body and may result in death. Still, drinking is considered socially acceptable in many parts because it is legal. Many people consider alcohol a stress reliever who wants to forget about the worries and tension of the day. However, as per a study, the fact is any amount of alcohol consumption is bad for health. If you are still not convinced, then read carefully below the most important reasons you should quit alcohol as early as you can.

Below are the Top 10 Reasons Why Alcohol is a Big No No:

1. Promotes Depression

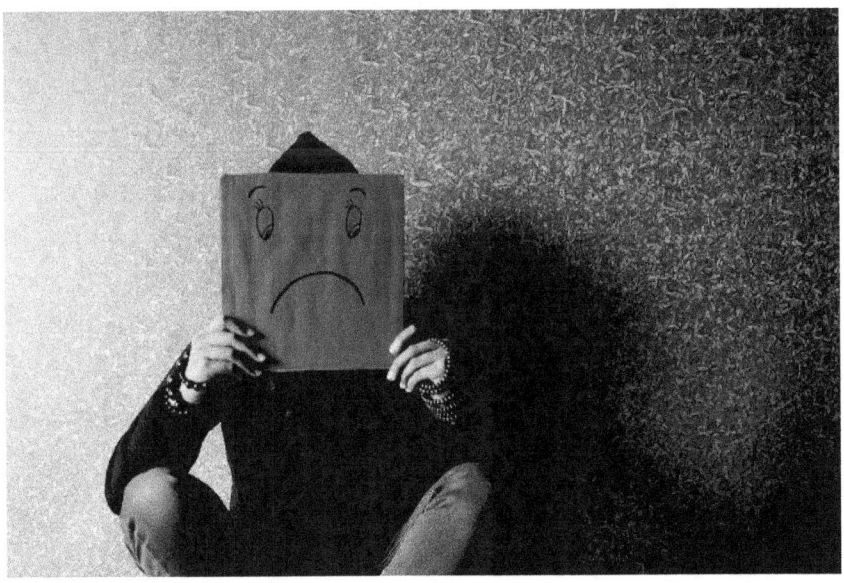

Are you worried about why you feel depressed all the time for every small issue? Alcohol is a direct central nervous system depressant that disrupts mood stability and promotes depression.

2. Brain Disorders

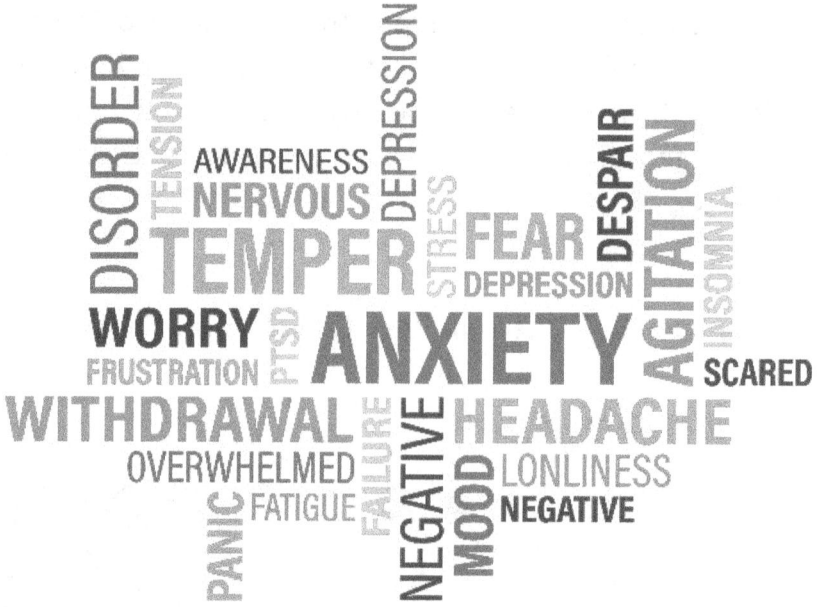

Alcohol interferes with the process of memory and affects the ability of new learning. Just one or two drinks are enough to cause slow reaction time, blurred vision, slow speech, impaired memory, and balance loss. These short-term effects disappear when you stop drinking alcohol, but prolonged alcohol consumption can cause neurological disorders that are severe and irreversible.

3. Cancer

International Agency for Research on Cancer (IARC) has classified alcoholic beverages as a Group 1 carcinogen (carcinogenic to humans). Drinking alcohol over extended periods is associated with a higher risk of certain types of cancer, including cancer of the mouth, throat, lung, esophagus, and breast. People who drink as well as smoke are at a higher risk of developing cancer. 3.6% of all cancer cases and 3.5% of cancer deaths worldwide are attributable to alcohol consumption (also known formally as ethanol).

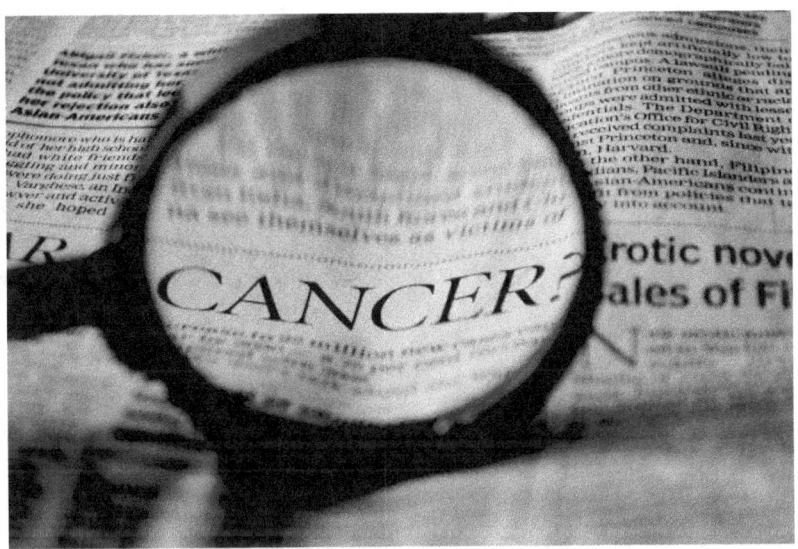

4. Weight Gain

Alcohol can cause weight gain in many ways:

- It is high in calories.
- It stops your body from burning fat.
- It can make you feel hungry.
- It can lead to unhealthy food choices.

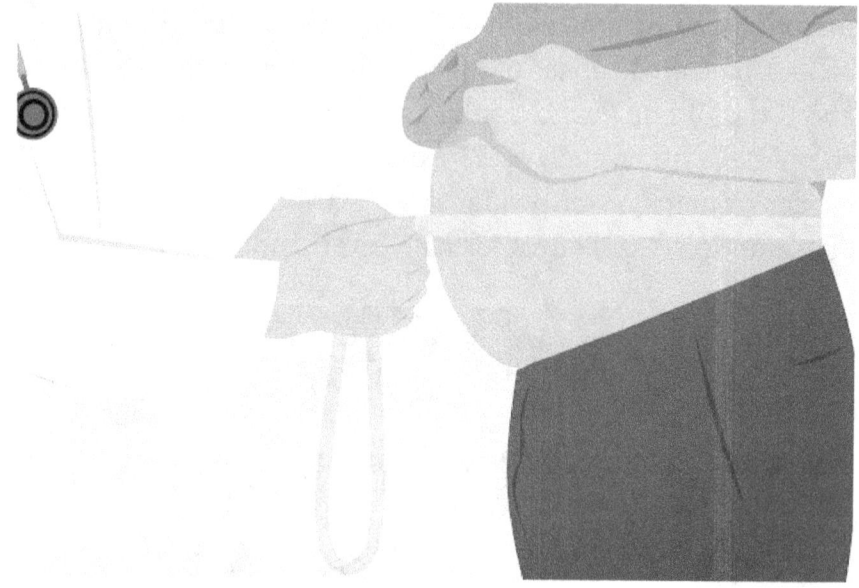

5.Risk of Injury

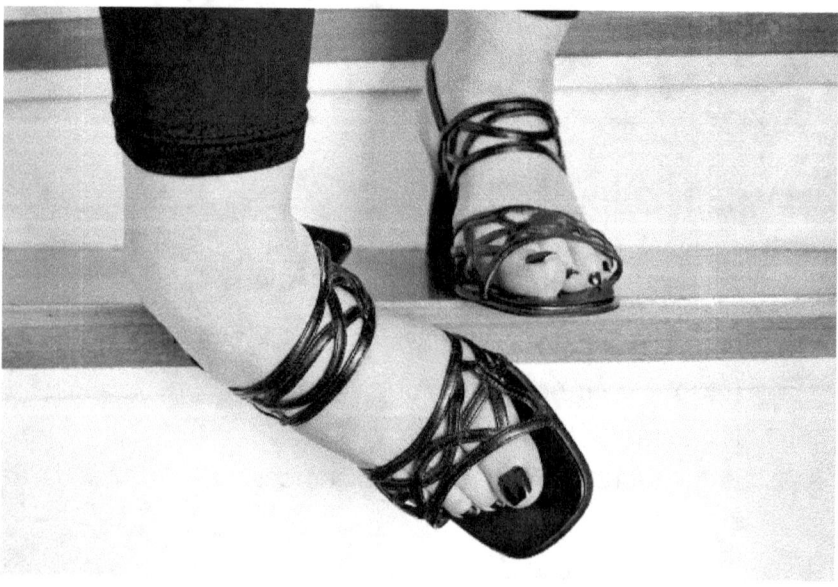

Alcoholic beverages slow the reaction time and impair judgment and coordination. People under the influence of alcohol are at higher risk for accidental injury.

6. Birth Defects

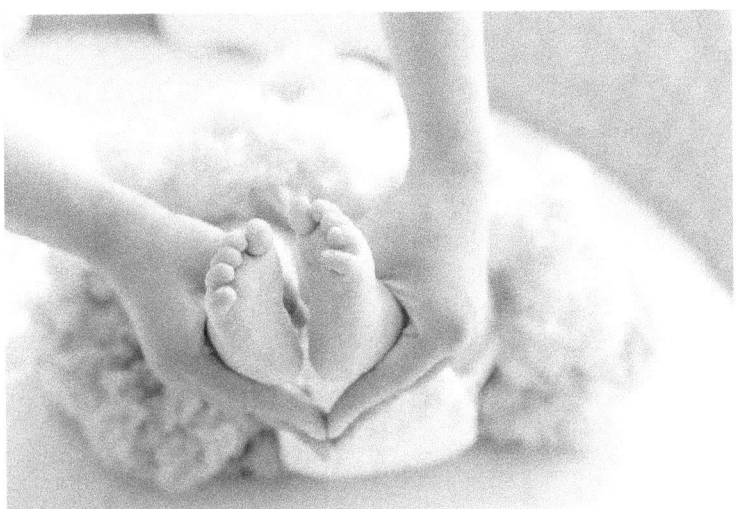

Pregnant women should not drink at all. Exposing the fetus to alcohol can cause defects of the brain, heart, and other organs in the baby. If a woman drinks alcohol while pregnant, the risk of giving birth to a child with fetal alcohol syndrome is very high. Fetal alcohol syndrome is a condition that affects the developing fetus. Children with fetal alcohol syndrome often have abnormal facial characteristics, stunted growth, organ defects, brain damage, and poor coordination. Fetal alcohol syndrome cannot be cured. Once the damage has been done to a child, he or she must suffer for life.

7. Cirrhosis of the Liver

Alcohol can lead to permanent organ damage. Liver cirrhosis can be fatal because the damaged liver cannot perform the essential processes required to keep the body functioning optimally. Cirrhosis affects the liver's ability to convert food into energy and prevent the removal of toxins from the body. When you have cirrhosis, your liver contains scar tissue that reduces blood flow through the organ. As a result, the liver cannot work effectively.

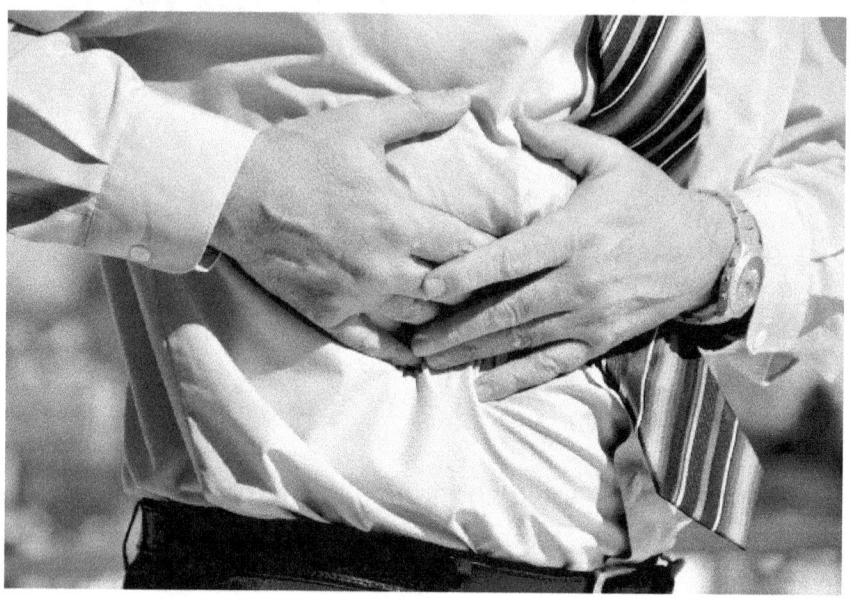

8. Serious Chronic Diseases

Long-term alcohol consumption can raise blood pressure and increase heart attack risk. Drinking too much alcohol can cause liver cirrhosis (damage to liver cells) and pancreatitis (inflammation of the pancreas).

9. Drug Interaction

Alcohol interferes with the therapeutic effect of the prescribed medication, including anti-depressant and anti-anxiety medications. It can be dangerous in combination with other medicines. Never take aspirin for alcoholic headaches. It can cause internal gastric bleeding, which can be life-threatening.

10. Abnormal Sleep Pattern

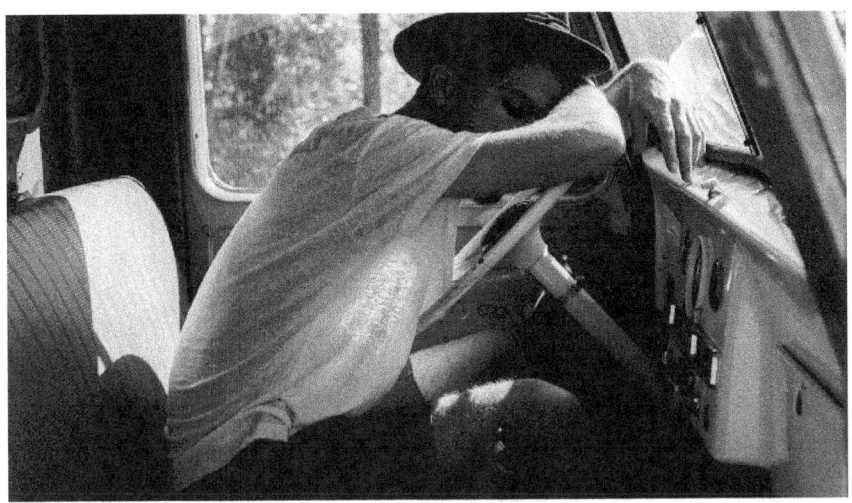

Alcohol interrupts the normal sleep pattern, which affects energy, mood, anxiety level. You feel tired all day.

My Thoughts

It is a misconception that you can enjoy your life with only a glass of alcoholic beverage. It is a human tendency to follow what he sees. It is not entirely our fault as we often see alcohol in movies and serials as a fun factor of life. They portray the most dangerous substance- alcohol as a cool thing or as a status symbol. But we should never forget that movies and serials are the pure art of fiction and have nothing to do with real life. Being a scientist, I have worked closely with alcohol. For me, alcohol is just another chemical substance that we use in a minimal amount to prepare tablets and capsules to treat a particular disease. We use a lesser quantity because we know how dangerous alcohol is to our body. You only live once; It is better to live your life disease-free, frustration-free, and depression-free. This is your fundamental right, do not let alcohol steal your basic living rights.

CHAPTER 3

10 SMART WAYS TO INCORPORATE PUMPKIN INTO YOUR DIET

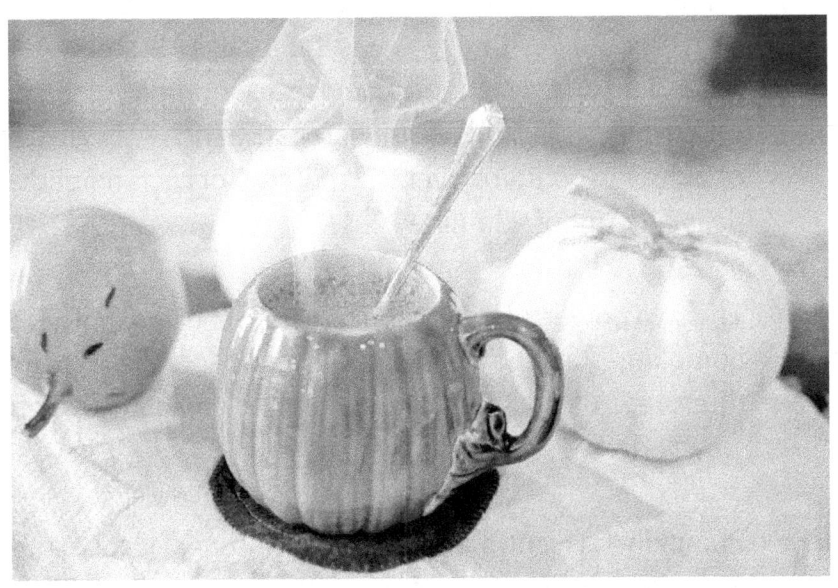

When I was a kid, my Mom used to chase me to make me eat pumpkin subji (curry) along with a long lecture on benefits of the pumpkin, but as a kid, I was not a fan of pumpkin. Yes, we all have been gone through this. I wish someone had told my Mom the smart ways to incorporate pumpkin in the diet like I am telling you today.

Before going into more detail, let's first see why pumpkin is so important to eat, especially if you are a student.

Benefits of Pumpkin:

- Pumpkin is high in vitamins and minerals while being low in calories as it's 94% water which makes pumpkin a weight-loss-friendly food.

- Pumpkin is rich in beta-carotene, a carotenoid that converts into vitamin A in the body. Vitamin A is essential for eyesight and helps the retina absorb and process light, making it a must for students. A single cup of pumpkin contains over 200 percent of recommended daily amount of vitamin A.

- The two powerful antioxidants, lutein and zeaxanthin in pumpkin, play the part of sunscreen for the eyes by filtering out the high-energy damaging light wavelengths.

- Pumpkin has antibacterial and antifungal properties. Pumpkin contains 20 percent of the recommended daily intake of vitamin C, which boosts your immunity and may help you recover from colds faster.

- Research suggests that a diet rich in beta-carotene can reduce the risk of prostate cancer.

Now we know how much pumpkin is important to our health. Below are 10 smart ways to incorporate pumpkin into your diet:

10 Smart Ways to Incorporate Pumpkin into Your Diet:

1. Pumpkin Oats Cake

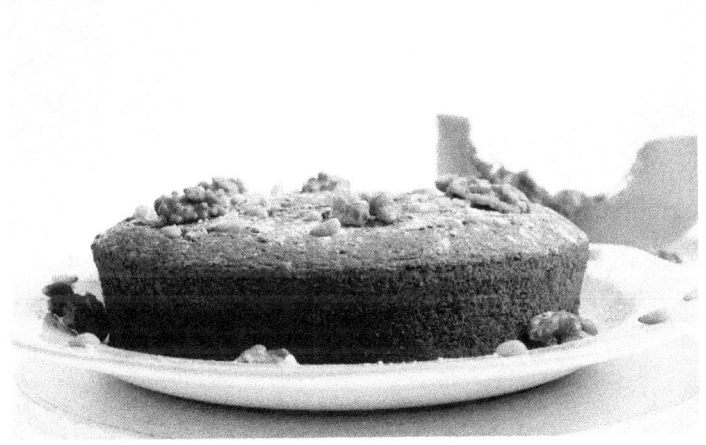

When you can't get your mind off dessert, try this healthier option. Instead of your regular cake, enjoy pumpkin and oats cake. Spiced with nutmeg and honey, 2-3 slices of this cake are enough to provide the required vitamin A for the entire day.

2. Pumpkin Halwa

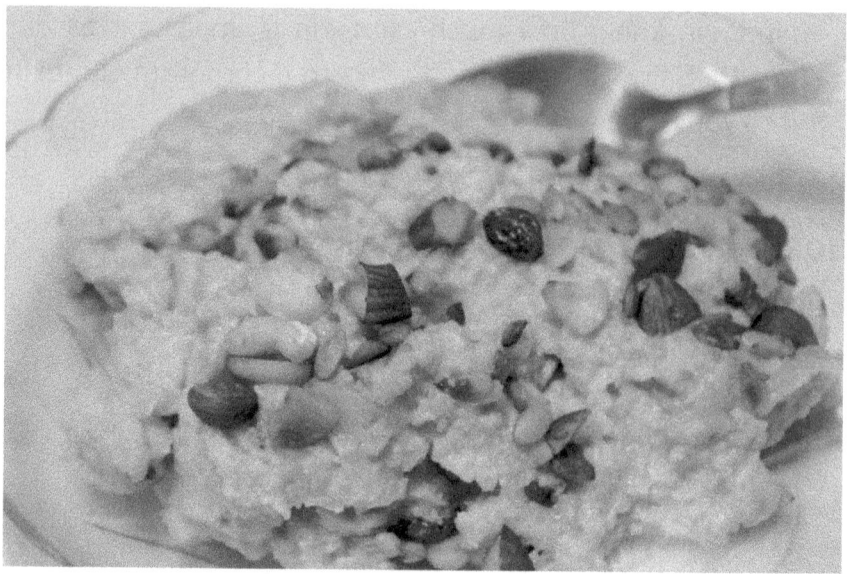

Give *gajar ka halwa* a rest for some time, and try this exotic pumpkin halwa this time. Top it off with some roasted desiccated coconut, almonds, and enjoy this dessert.

3. Roasted Pumpkin

A winner for everyone at the dinner table – bake pumpkin pieces and spice them up with peri-peri masala.

4. Pumpkin Coconut Cookie

Give your regular coconut cookies a twist, add some grated pumpkin along with coconut, and enjoy your healthier cookie.

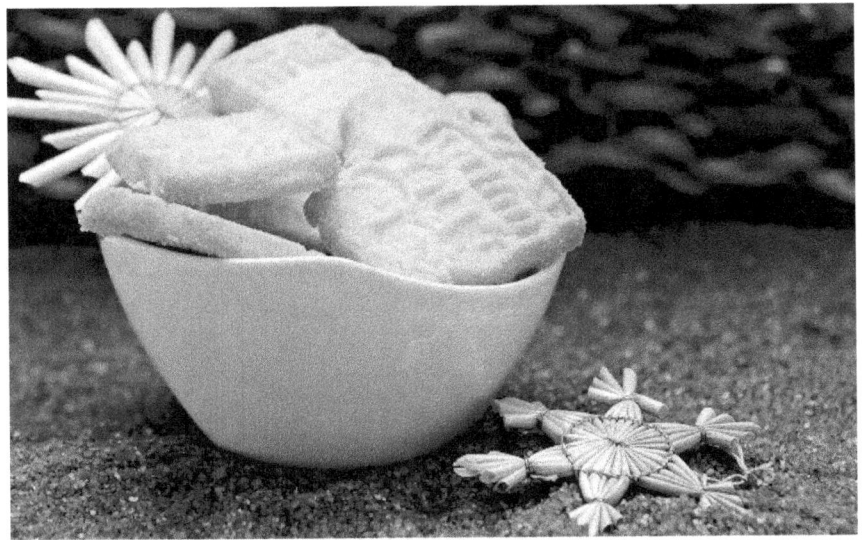

5. Pumpkin Masala Thepla

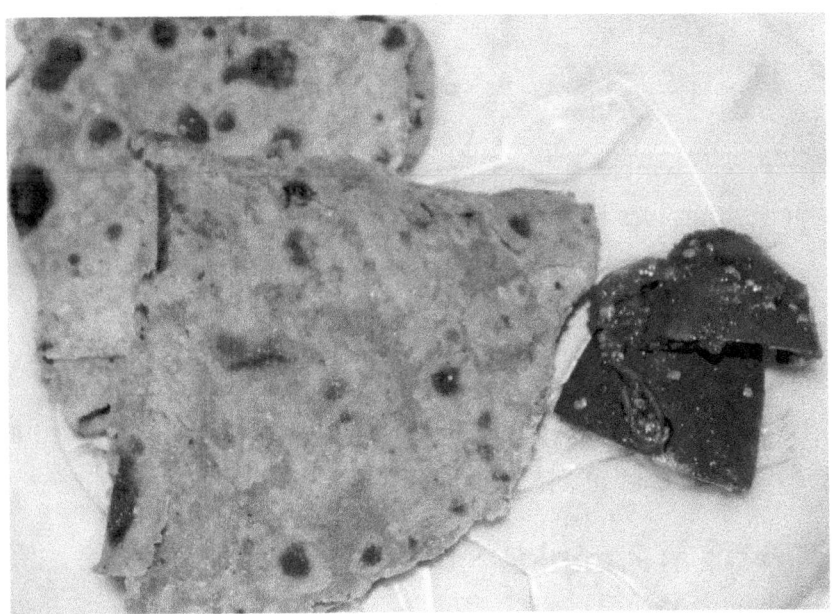

This one is my favorite. Add some grated pumpkin to your regular masala thepla, and enjoy this breakfast dish.

6. Whole-Grain Pumpkin Pancakes

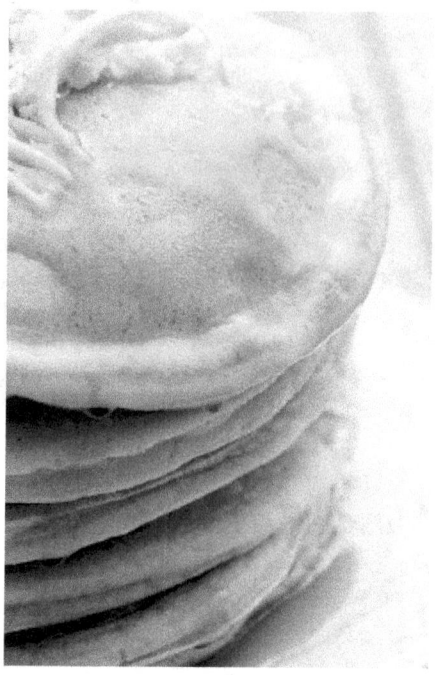

Perfect for winter, this hearty breakfast recipe includes whole-wheat flour, lots of spices, pumpkin, and milk.

7. Pumpkin Tikki

Grate some pumpkin and other veggies. Add some boiled potatoes and herbs of your choice. Roll it in breadcrumbs, shallow fry them, and enjoy with tomato sauce.

8. Pasta in Pumpkin Sauce

Creamy pasta dishes are often full of fat and cholesterol. Instead of making your dinner a giant calorie bomb, try pumpkin cream sauce and use Greek yogurt instead of heavy cream to make your pasta tastier and healthier.

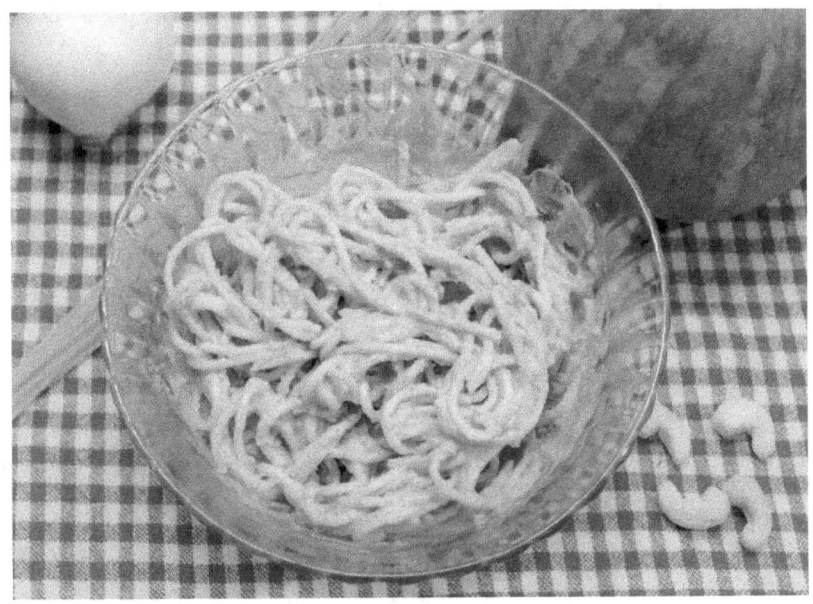

9. Pumpkin Almond Muffins

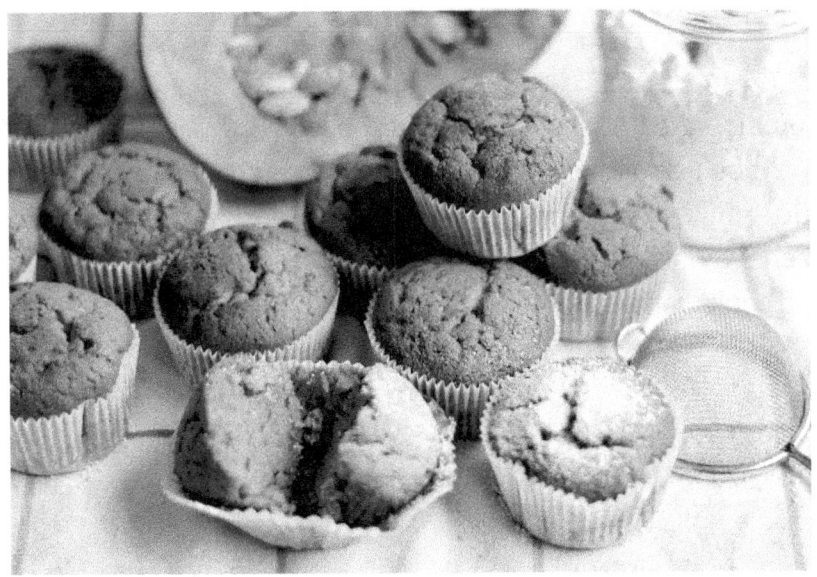

Start your day with pumpkin almond muffins. These mouth-watering muffins make for a perfect snack on-the-go and will keep you going until it's time for lunch.

10. Pumpkin Waffles

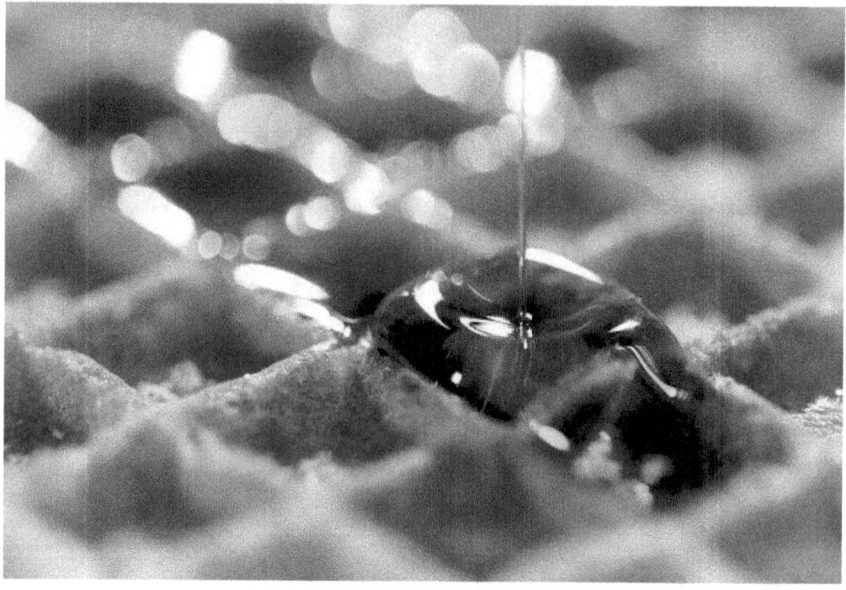

Combine the flour, sugar, baking soda, baking powder, and salt in a bowl and stir well. Add the wet ingredients: pumpkin, buttermilk, butter, and vanilla essence, and mix until smooth. Preheat waffle iron. Brush the waffle iron with melted butter and cook waffles. Eat with toppings of your choice.

My Thoughts

If you don't like pumpkins just like me but still want to eat them because of their health benefits, then these were my ideas of smartly incorporating pumpkin in the diet, which will be tasty yet healthy. And if you are already a Pumpkin lover, then you got some more interesting recipes on your list.

CHAPTER 4

PREVENTION IS ACTUALLY BETTER THAN CURE

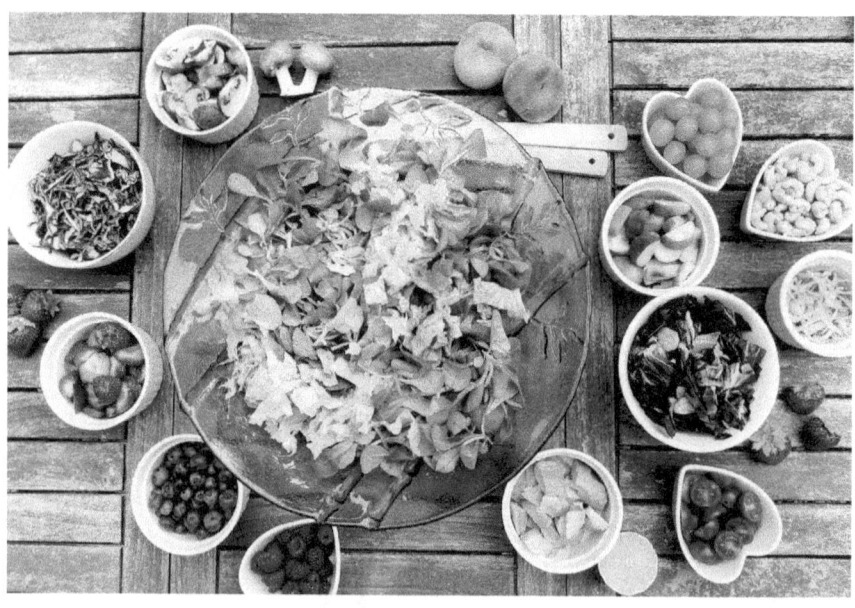

We all know *Prevention is Better Than Cure* but how many of us apply it in our life? The percentage is very low. Generally, when we see someone having a consequence of their bad habits, we assume that it can only happen to others. We tend to think harmful consequences only happen to others; somewhere, we believe we are different; this will definitely not happen to me. But the fact is no matter if you irresponsibly behave toward your health today, it is coming back to you sooner or later; there is no escape.

I know I am sounding harsh, but that's the fact. The simple rule is that what you give to your body, your body will give you the same in response. Therefore, if you are giving junk, health deteriorating elements to your body, then you should not expect a healthy life in return. Sometimes our body does not immediately alarm for junk and bad habits, and everything seems very normal, but over time, it aggregates, and then it gives you life-threatening illnesses. After all, our body needs good care, good foods, a good lifestyle, and when the body does not get it, its function gets affected, and over time it loses its functionality.

I see many people talking about their health problems as if God has given them these problems. They do not even consider thinking or analyzing whether they have done something wrong that has caused them this particular health problem. I believe prevention is better than cure. You have to analyze what is this health problem, what is the root cause of it, is it due to your poor eating habits or poor bad lifestyle choices? What exactly went wrong?

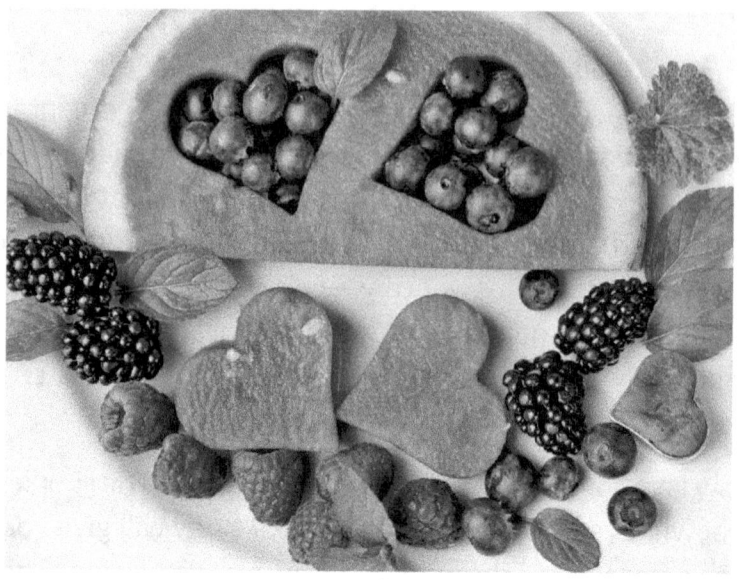

We know that stress causes health problems. If I ask you to think the opposite way? What if I tell you that if you have a health problem, you will be stressed due to your health problem. If you are not feeling healthy, how will you focus on other important aspects of your life? Won't you lose major opportunities in your life because of your health problems?

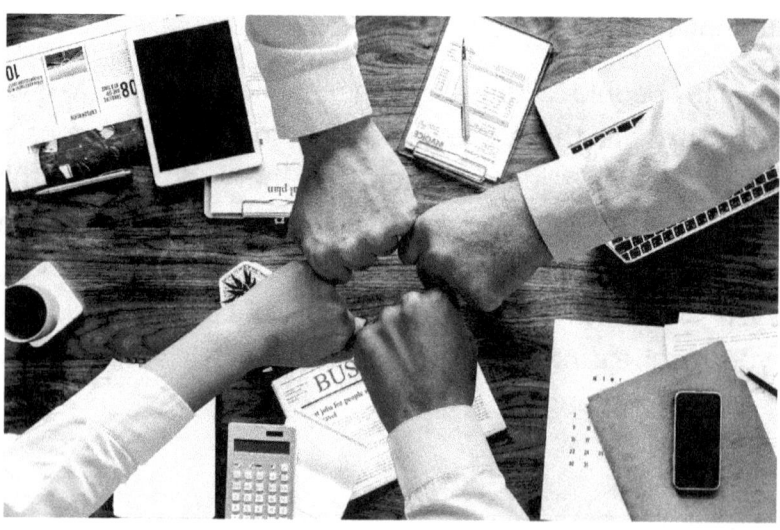

See in this way, if this helps you, God has gifted you this body, you are the caretaker of your body, everything else will come and go, but your body will remain with you for the lifetime.

If you are responsible for anything most, then it is your body. If you will not fulfill your responsibility, then who else will be?

Conclusion

At last, all I can say that your body is not a dustbin where you can throw anything. It is the temple; you should worship it and think twice before giving it any junk or health deterioration elements. Because ultimately, what you will give to your body, it will give you back the same.

CHAPTER 5

RECIPES

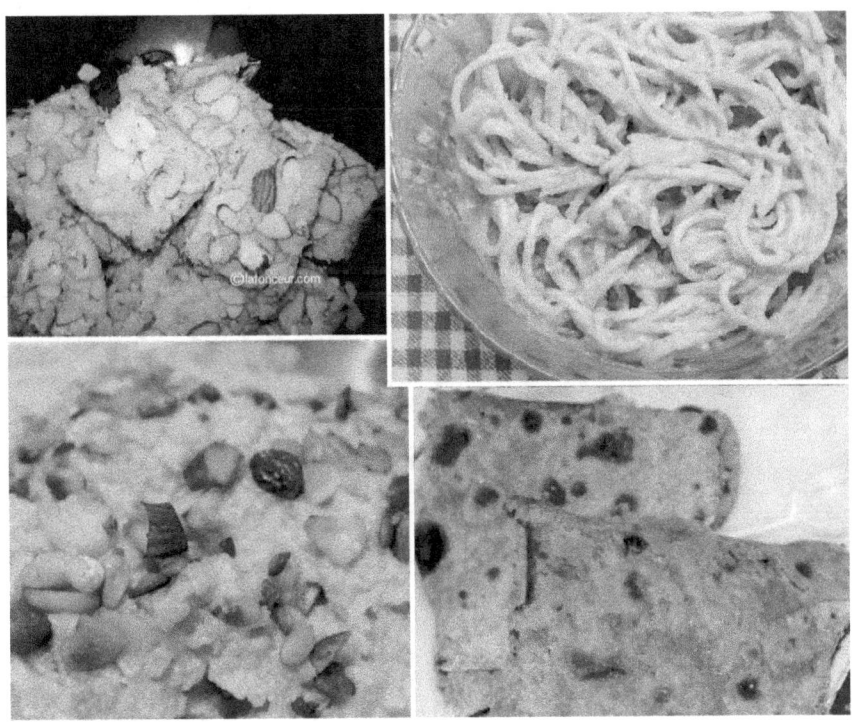

Coconut Burfi Sweet and Healthy

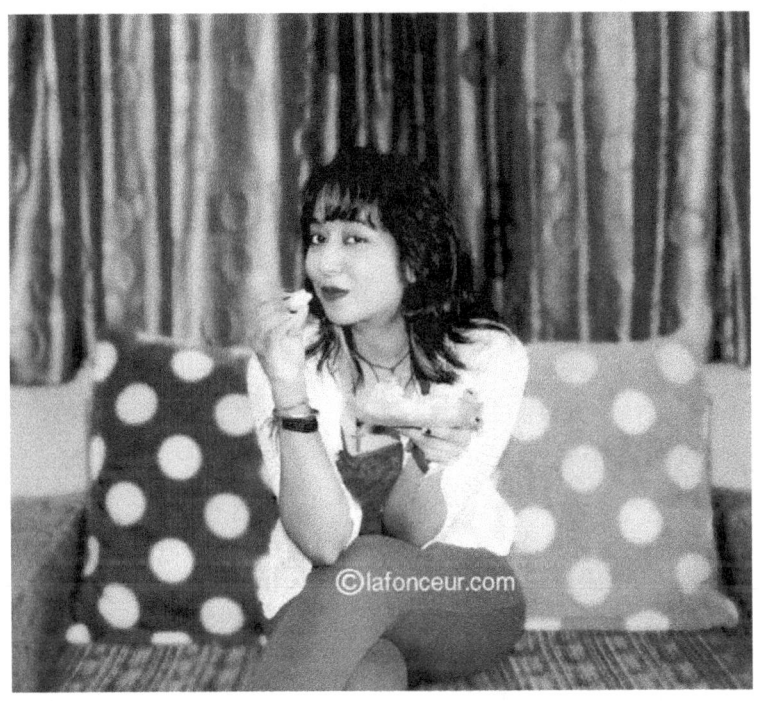

C oconut burfi is healthy as it has nuts. You can make it even healthier by substituting refined white sugar with brown sugar. If you substitute use jaggery instead of brown sugar, it would be even more beneficial to health. Also, replace normal unsalted butter with **ghee** (clarified butter made from cow's milk).

If you are health conscious but sweet tooth, then coconut burfi is the best option you can go for without even second thought.

Health Benefits of Coconut Burfi:

Desiccated coconut:

We all know coconut contains fat but healthy fat, which is essential for body function. It lowers LDL levels (bad cholesterol) and increases good cholesterol or HDL, strengthening your arteries and promoting cardiovascular health. Other than that, it is very good for the skin and helps in the brain's better functioning. It contains several essential nutrients, including dietary fiber, manganese, copper, and selenium.

Cow Ghee (Unsalted clarified butter):

As per Ayurved, cow Ghee is very good for health. Cow ghee is full of essential nutrients, healthy fats and has antibacterial, antifungal, antioxidants, and antiviral properties. It normalizes Vata and Pitta and nourishes the body. It is known as a brain tonic. Excellent for improving memory power and intelligence. Best for strengthening mental health. It is beneficial for curing thyroid dysfunction. It heals wounds, chapped lips, and mouth ulcers and best for joints' lubrication. It cures insomnia. But it should consume in moderation if you don't want to put on weight.

Jaggery:

Jaggery boosts immunity. The ability to purify the blood is the most well-known of all the benefits of jaggery. Jaggery is among the best natural cleansing agents for the body. It Prevents anemia, controls blood pressure, and prevents respiratory problems. Jaggery has a complex carbohydrate that gives energy to the body gradually and for a longer time, therefore, helps in preventing fatigue and weakness of the body.

How to make Coconut Burfi

Ingredients:
Desiccated coconut: 2 cups
Cow ghee (Unsalted clarified butter): 1 tablespoon
Cow's milk: 2 cups
Brown sugar/Jaggery: 3/4 cup
Saffron: a pinch
Shredded almond: For decoration

Method:

Soak saffron in 2 tablespoons of hot milk. Keep aside. Dry roast desiccated coconut.

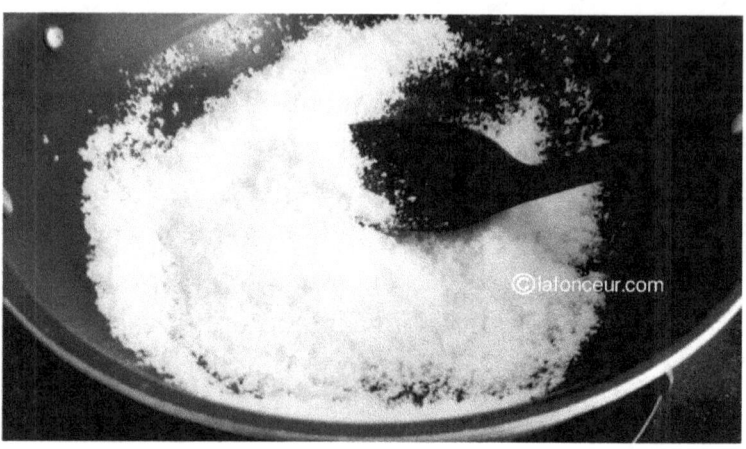

Heat 1 tablespoon Cow Ghee (Unsalted clarified butter).

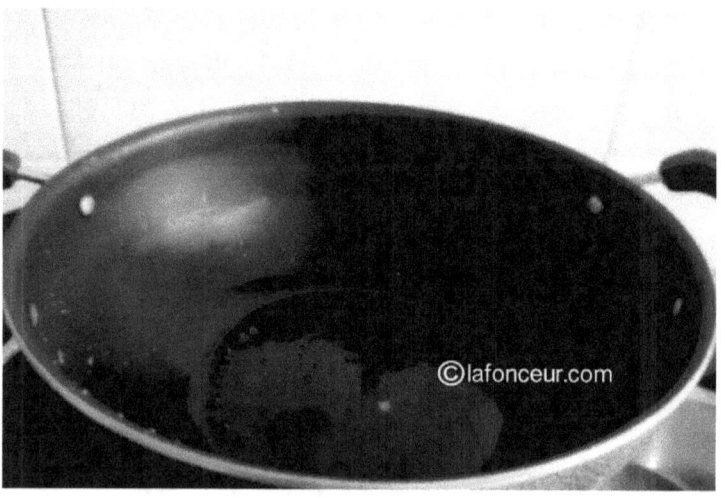

Add cow's milk.

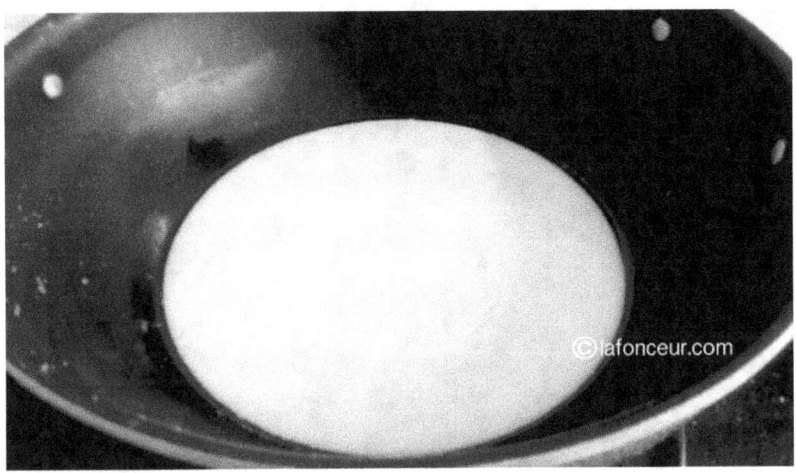

Bring it to a boil and reduce it to half.

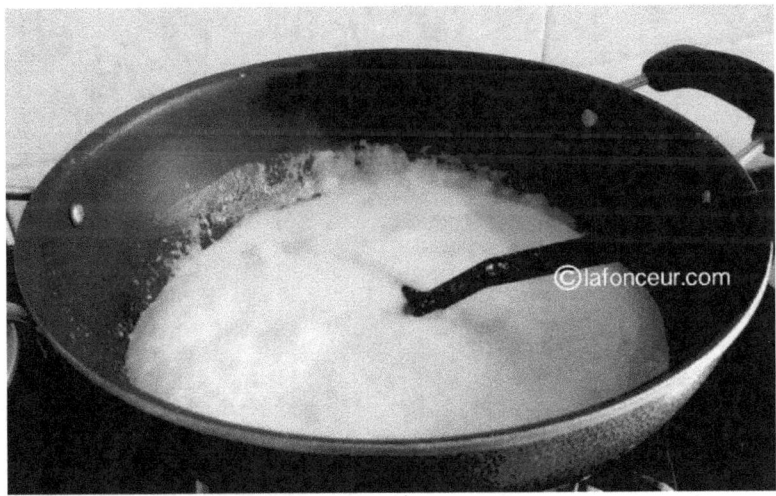

Add brown sugar or jaggery.

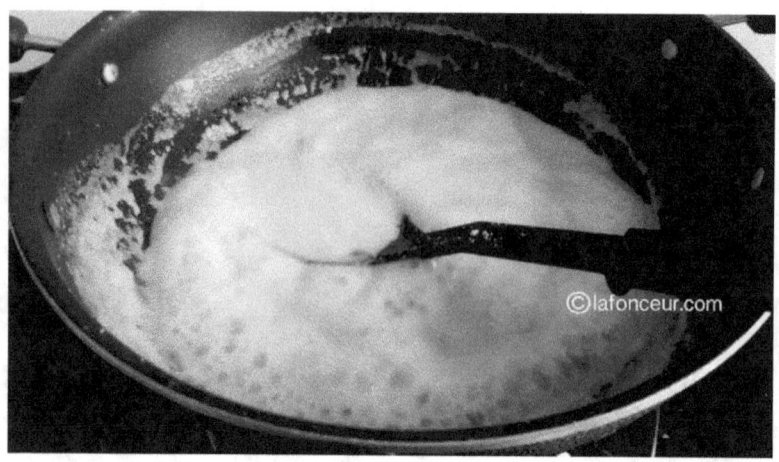

Add roasted desiccated coconut.

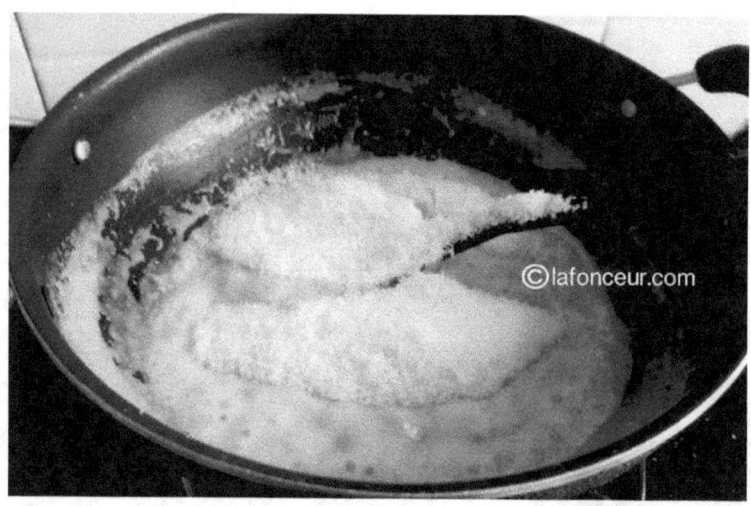

and mix well.

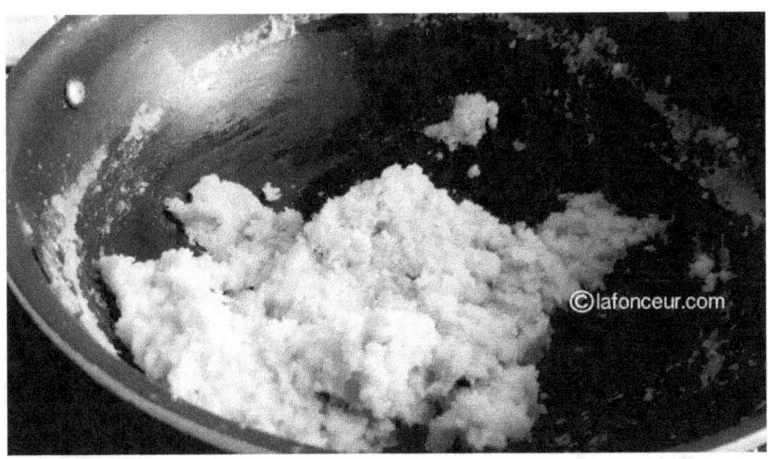

Add saffron soaked in milk.

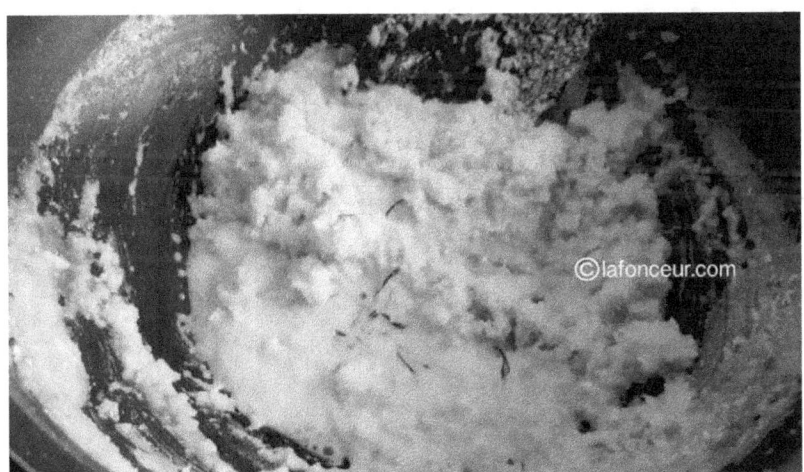

Pour it into a baking dish.

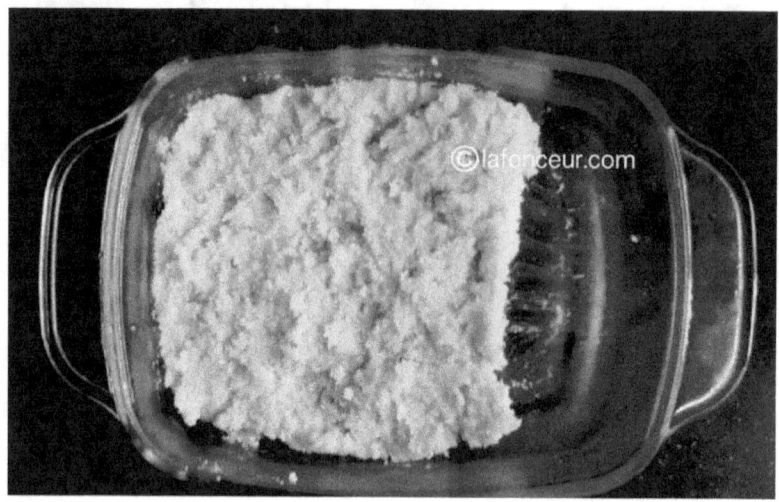

Sprinkle shredded almond and cut them into squares.

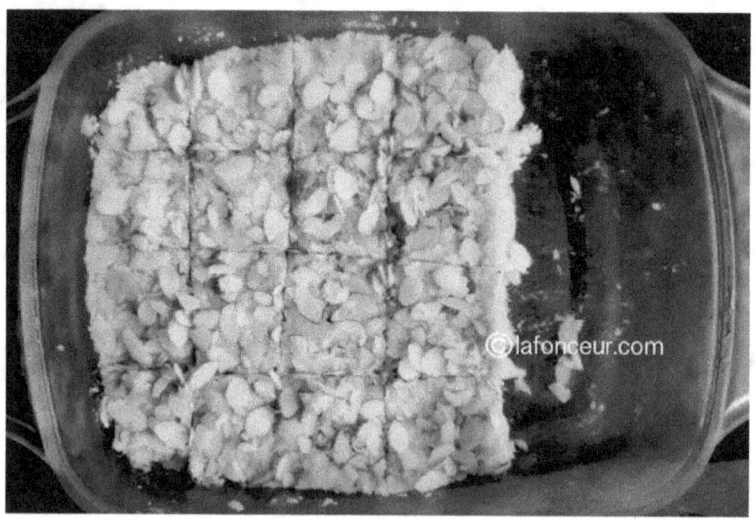

Refrigerate for 2 hours and voila Coconut Burfi is ready to eat.

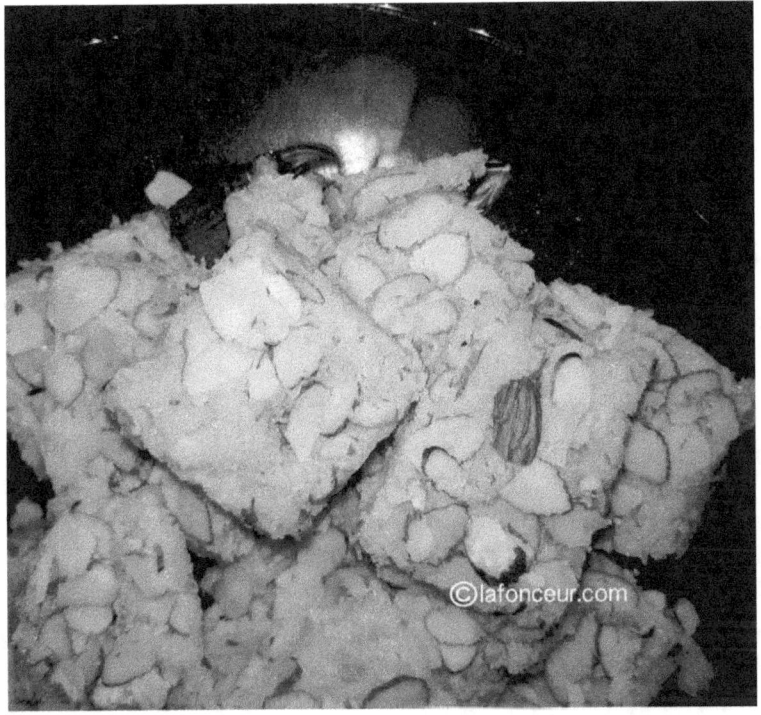

The best part of coconut burfi is you can consume it without worrying about your health. Do try yourself to satisfy your sweet craving.

Spaghetti in Creamy Pumpkin Sauce

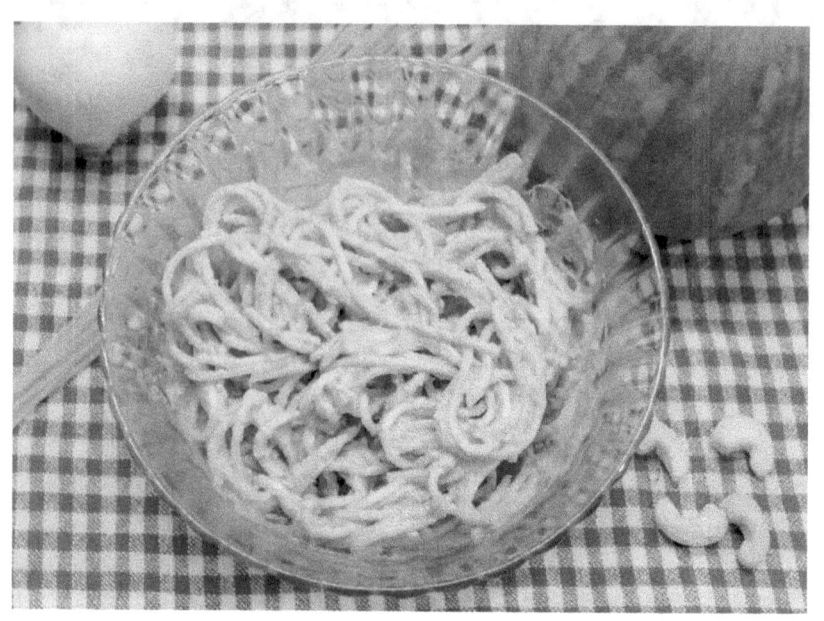

<u>Serves: 2</u>

Ingredients:

Cooked spaghetti: 200 gm

Pumpkin: 300 gm

Cashew nuts: ½ cup

Garlic: 5 cloves

White onion: 1 large

Red chili powder: ½ teaspoon

Black pepper: a pinch

Salt: To taste

Water: 1 cup

Olive oil: 2 tablespoons

Method:

<u>For Pumpkin Puree</u>

1. Take a pressure cooker. Add roughly chopped pumpkin and ½ cup water. Add salt. Pressure cook for 2 whistles.

2. Mash the pumpkin with a spatula.

<u>For Pumpkin Sauce</u>

1. Soak cashew nuts in ½ cup hot water for 15-20 mins. Drain the water and keep the soaked cashew nuts aside.

2.Take a pan. Add 2 tablespoons of olive oil. Heat it. Crush the garlic and immediately add it to the oil. Cook for 5 mins.

3. Add roughly chopped onion. Cook for 5-7 mins.

4. Add cashew nuts and cook for 3-5 mins.

5. Add pumpkin puree. Add red chili powder, black pepper, and salt (we have added salt in pumpkin puree too, so add accordingly).

6. Mix well. Cover the mixture with a lid and cook at low flame

for 10-15 mins. Mix in between so that the mixture doesn't stick to the bottom of the pan.

7. Turn off the flame and let the mix cool. Now blend until very smooth with ¼ cup of water. The sauce should be smooth, thick, and free from any lumps.

8. Take out the sauce in a bowl. Add spaghetti and mix well. Your creamy and healthy spaghetti is ready to eat.

Note:

1. Crush garlic just before adding it to oil for enhanced garlic flavor.

2. Cook the pumpkin mix with the lid on for at least 10 mins to remove the raw taste of pumpkin and onion.

3. Use white onion because white onions are sweeter and milder than yellow and purple onion.

4. The smoother you blend the creamer will be your pumpkin sauce.

Pumpkin Halwa

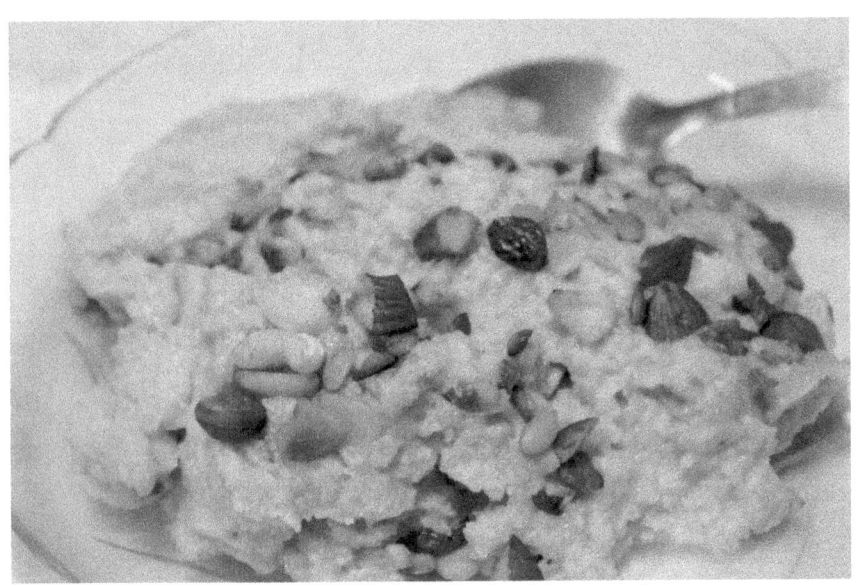

Ingredients:

Grated pumpkin: 500 gm

Milk: 500 ml

Almonds: 10-12

Cashew nuts: 10-12

Raisins 10-12

Melon seeds: 1 tablespoon

Jaggery: 100 gm or Brown sugar: ½ cup

Desiccated coconut: 3 tablespoons

Ghee: 1 teaspoon

Method:

1. Take a deep pan. Add milk and bring it to a boil.

2. Add grated pumpkin. Cook on medium-high flame for 15 min.

3. Meanwhile, chop almonds and cashew nuts. Take 1 teaspoon of ghee in another pan and heat it. Add almonds, cashew nuts, melon seeds, and raisins.

4. Sauté the nuts and seeds till they start releasing an aromatic smell and turn slightly brown. Remove the nuts from heat. Store in an air-tight container.

5. After 15 min the pumpkin and milk mixture will turn into a thick paste. Add jaggery and desiccated coconut at this stage.

6. Cook the halwa for another 10 min till it starts leaving the pan.

7. Turn off the flame. Let the pumpkin halwa cool. Refrigerate it for 2 hours. Sprinkle the nuts just before serving and enjoy this healthy and tasty dessert.

Pumpkin Masala Thepla

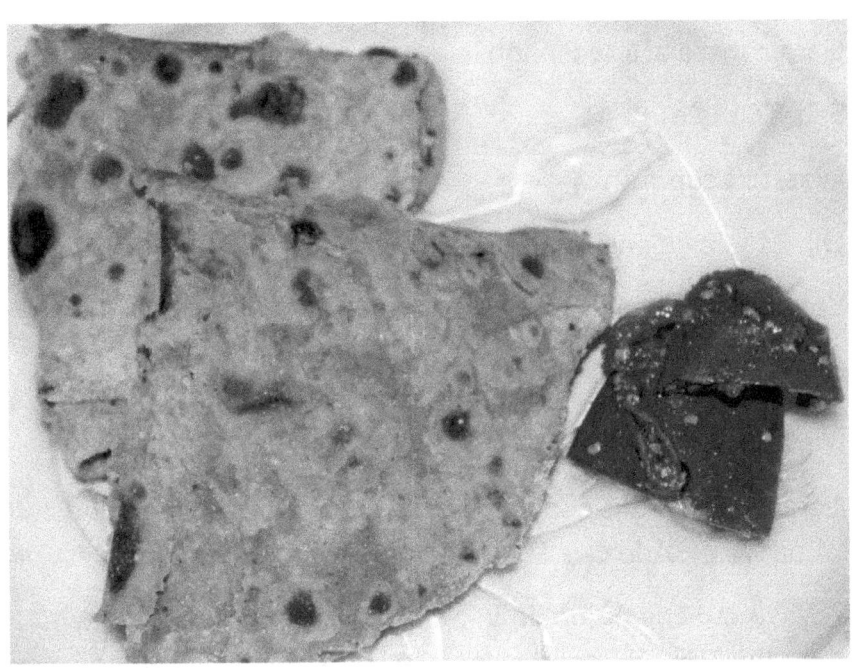

<u>Serves: 2</u>

Ingredients:

Pumpkin: 300 gm

Whole wheat flour: 1 cup

Millet flour: ½ cup

Chickpea flour: ½ cup

Turmeric powder: ½ teaspoon

Grated ginger: 1 tablespoon

Chopped green chilies: 1 teaspoon

White sesame seeds: 1 teaspoon

Garam masala: 1 teaspoon

Salt: To taste

Water: ½ cup

Oil: 3 tablespoons

Yogurt: 2 tablespoons (If required)

Method

1. Take a pressure cooker. Add roughly chopped pumpkin and ½ cup water. Add salt. Pressure cook for 2 whistles.

2. Take out the pumpkin in a bowl. Mash the pumpkin with a spatula. Add all the rest of the ingredients except oil and yogurt.

3. Knead to a soft dough. Pumpkin has high water content, plus we have added water while making the puree, so no additional water is required for kneading. But if your dough looks dry, add 1 to 2 tablespoons of thick yogurt.

4. Divide the dough into 8-9 equal parts. Make medium-sized dough balls.

5. Take one piece of the dough ball, dip it in the dry whole wheat flour, and dust off the excess flour.

6. Use a rolling pin to roll the dough into a thin 5 inch-6 inch circle.

7. Heat the pan/griddle (tawa) on medium-high flame.

8. Place the thepla on the griddle. Cook for about a minute or cook until the thepla begins puffing up from the base at some places.

9. Flip the thepla and spread 3-4 drops of oil. Cook for 2 minutes until it turns light brown.

10. Flip the thepla again and top with 3-4 drops of oil, spreading it evenly over the surface. Gently press the thepla with the flat spatula to help it cook evenly.

11. Once brown spots are visible on both sides of the thepla, transfer it to a serving plate. Similarly, make all the theplas.

12. Enjoy pumpkin masala thepla with pickle of your choice in breakfast.

READ THE COMPLETE SERIES

Read the complete Eat So What! Mini Editions Series:

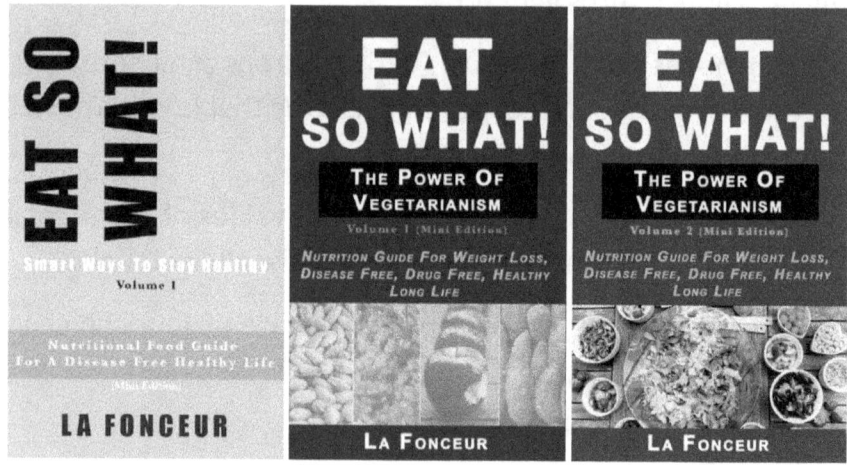

| Book 1 | Book 3 | Book 4 |

ABOUT THE AUTHOR

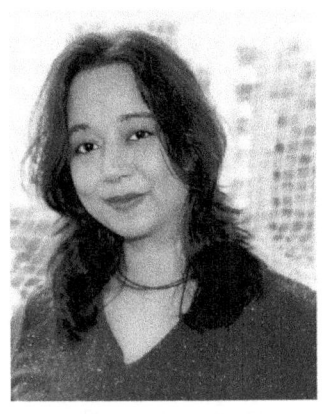

La Fonceur is the author of the book series **Eat So What!**, **Secret of Healthy Hair**, and **Eat to Prevent and Control Disease.** She is a health blogger and a dance artist. She has a master's degree in Pharmacy. She specialized in Pharmaceutical Technology and worked as a research scientist in the research and development department. She has published an article titled "Techniques for Producing Biotechnology-Derived Products of Pharmaceutical Use" in the Pharmtechmedica Journal. She is also a registered pharmacist. Being a research scientist, she has worked closely with drugs. Based on her experience, she believes that one can prevent most diseases with nutritious vegetarian foods and a healthy lifestyle.

NOTE FROM LA FONCEUR

Dear Reader,

Thank you for reading *Eat So What! Smart Ways to Stay Healthy Volume 2*. I hope you have found this book helpful.

If you liked the book, please leave a short review online telling why you enjoyed reading it. This will help other health-conscious readers find this book. Your help in spreading awareness is gratefully received.

Join my mailing list at www.eatsowhat.com/esw-newsletter to receive updates on my new release.

———————————————————

Also, read how foods that work with the same mechanism as medicines can naturally prevent and control disease in *Eat to Prevent and Control Disease*.

If you are looking for a permanent solution to your hair problems, read *Secret of Healthy Hair*.

All of my books are available in eBook, paperback, and hardcover editions. Happy reading!

Regards

La Fonceur

ALL BOOKS BY LA FONCEUR

Full-length books:

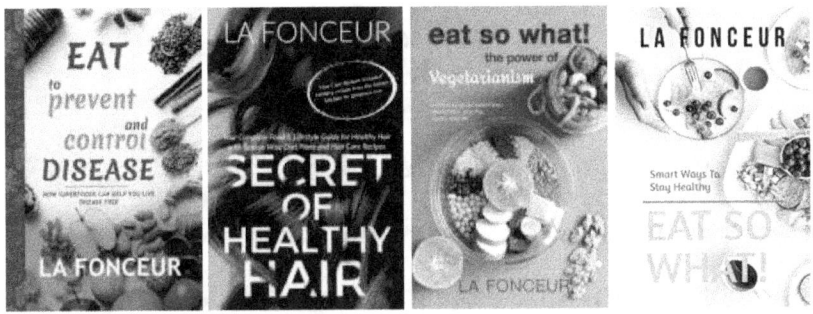

Mini extract editions:

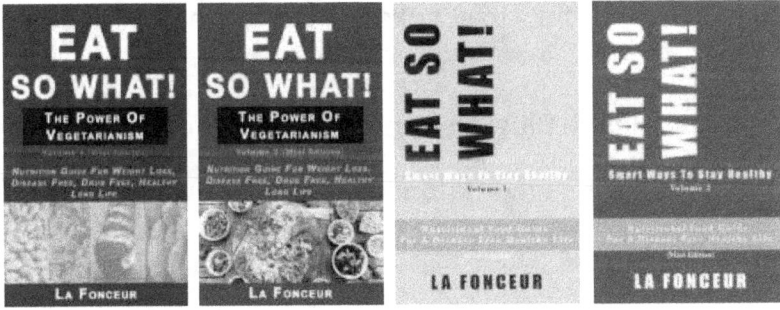

Hindi editions:

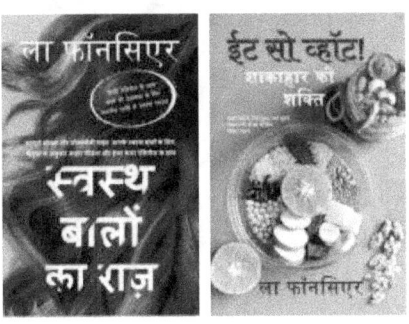

CONNECT WITH LA FONCEUR

Instagram: **@la_fonceur** | **@eatsowhat**

Facebook: **LaFonceur** | **eatsowhat**

Twitter: **@la_fonceur**

Amazon Author Page:

www.amazon.com/La-Fonceur/e/B07PM8SBSG/

Bookbub: **www.bookbub.com/authors/la-fonceur**

Sign up to the websites to get exclusive offers on La Fonceur eBooks:

Health Blog: **www.eatsowhat.com**

Website: **www.lafonceur.com/sign-up**

www.ingramcontent.com/pod-product-compliance
Lightning Source LLC
Chambersburg PA
CBHW072116280526
45788CB00006B/2527